# Inspiring True Stories of Everyday Heroes

From the Frontlines of #COVID-19

Cover Design: Ronda Taylor, heartworkcreative.com

ISBN: 978-1-7359748-8-0
E-Book ISBN: 978-1-7359748-9-7

Published by: The Unapologetic Voice House
www.theunapologeticvoicehouse.com

*This book is dedicated to every essential worker and frontline hero who worked and continues to work through COVID-19.*

# Contents

# Introduction

THIS BOOK STARTED AS A PASSION PROJECT OF MINE. IT was exactly 30 days before my wedding when an executive order for the entire state of Arizona came down that prohibited gatherings of more than 10 people.

After talking with our wedding coordinator and securing a new date in eight months, I sent out an email to our 150 guests with brand new information.

Millions of soon-to-be-brides had to send an email out like that.

Our situation wasn't unique by any means. I mean, besides the fact that the love of my life has lung issues and is missing his spleen. COVID took that original wedding date from me, which in the big scheme of things isn't really anything. Still, it created some sadness and grief.

And being the CEO of The Unapologetic Voice House, I felt the calling to turn my sadness into something positive.

Within a few days of Arizona receiving the next executive order to stay at home, I decided to create this anthology book giving essential workers and frontline heroes the space to share their stories.

We've all seen images of nurses and doctors on Instagram pleading with us to wear our masks.

The lines of their PPE is so deeply embedded on their face.

They are mentally, physically and emotionally exhausted. They are scared and at their breaking point.

Meanwhile, we haven't seen our newborn baby nieces or nephews, our elderly parents, extended family, friends, teachers or colleagues for months.

We became homeschool teachers. Unemployed. Experts at online meetings. Confused.

And yet through it all, our gratitude to those who continue to support and serve is immense. There are so many stories from frontline heroes in your community.

Here are just a few.

Thank you for giving these heroes your time and energy.

Sincerely,

Carrie Severson

CEO

The Unapologetic Voice House

# My Journey of Hope

Cyndi Searles

S HE WAS TURNING 103 YEARS-OLD, BUT HER FAMILY could not be there with her. The staff and employees were all wearing masks, and gowns, and face shields, and gloves. She was sitting at a table alone, eating a cupcake, when I walked into this new, uncertain way of working as a nurse during the COVID-19 pandemic. This was my first experience in the New Jersey facility where I had voluntarily gone to offer help. And I immediately wondered what I had gotten myself into.

The residents were not allowed to interact with one another, in fact, they were required to stay in their rooms. Which meant that most of them were left in their beds because they were not able to walk on their own. The dining hall that once was bustling with activity, now sat empty. The hallways which were normally filled with people walking and in wheelchairs, and where voices and conversations could be heard, were now silent. Where once there were kind smiles, and warm touches, and time spent with each other, there was now limited touch and fear, or at least the uncertainty of catching a virus we were all unsure of.

It seemed that our entire world had changed overnight; and as time went on, we all wondered if it would ever go back to how things were. We watched the news and became more and more fearful every day. We watched the numbers increase day by day, and even watched the death toll rise in a way that had not been seen before. The sound of COVID-19 put a chill down the backs of almost everyone.

At first, I watched with the rest of the world as the number of infected people rose. I listened, trying to make sense of this new strain, and wondered what would become of it. I continued to work at my clinic in Arizona as we made changes to reflect the current situation. Even with all the changes and uncertainty, I was still thankful that I had a job after so many others had been laid off or asked to quit working. I watched as things became increasingly difficult in New York and New Jersey where there were so many people suffering and the death numbers kept rising. Then one day, I heard the call for help, the continued call for nurses, doctors, and other health care workers to help out in this time of crisis.

And then I thought, "What if I went to help?" "What if I left my comfort zone?" "What if I did this totally crazy thing?" I began to see how I could be useful, and I began to envision myself there, and I began to feel that it was my calling. And so, despite my fear and my anxiety and worry of what could happen, I answered the call to leave my husband and three kids in Arizona and go to New Jersey alone to help those on the front lines fighting some unknown enemy that appeared determined to take us out.

On April 25th, 2020, I said my tearful goodbyes at the quiet and desolate airport and wondered if I would see them again. And, if I would see them again, whether they would be healthy. I also wondered that I wouldn't recognize them if things changed so much. I feared I was getting into something I might not be able to handle, and I feared that I would be miserable and overwhelmed and all alone on the other side of the country where I didn't know anyone. With all these fears and uncertainties, I boarded the plane anyway; and I am so thankful that I did.

A few hours later, I stepped into the unknown. Without knowing where or if I would land, I took that first giant leap into the darkness, trusting and hoping that I would not only survive, but that I would become even stronger from my experiences. As I watched the 103 year old woman tell the staff why she should get the first cupcake, I looked out at the flag flying at half-mast, and saw her family spread out on the lawn holding up a sign that read, "Happy 103rd Birthday!" I realized then that everything had changed. These are some stories from my experience on the front lines as a nurse, and I wouldn't change a thing!

## Elliot

Elliot was a very confused resident who loved to eat and looked out for his roommate. He didn't speak much, but he understood a lot of what was said. He had become incontinent, so he wore adult briefs and, most days, he wore a hospital gown because that was the easiest thing for him to keep on. He loved to wander the halls and did not understand the quarantine orders or what was going on. Very often, he would be up and down the hallway. He wore a baseball cap most of the time and had an enlarged belly. I can just picture him in his cap and hospital gown that was completely open at the back with his adult brief on, and he would just scratch an itch on his butt or private parts without a care in the world. It was quite humorous at times. Trying to get him to keep his oxygen tubing in his nose became a whole new issue when he became positive with COVID-19 and began to have trouble breathing.

## Mary

Mary was a sweet, elderly woman with kind eyes. She would reach out her hand and loved to take my hand and put it up to her face. She would touch my face shield and ask why I had it on, and she would often start crying and state, "Don't leave me, please don't leave me!" And when I would ask her what was wrong, she would just cry harder. I would sit with her for a few minutes when I could, and just hold her hand and stroke her hair even though she had tested positive for COVID-19. I knew I was potentially putting myself at risk by being with her for any longer than I medically needed to be near her. She would thank me later and tell me that she appreciated the time I gave her. She was one of the fortunate ones who survived the virus.

## Anthony

Anthony required feedings and medications to be given through a tube that fed into his stomach. One day, I went into his room to give him his feeding, and he said to me, "So when are we getting married?" I laughed and told him that I would need to check with my husband before I could answer his question. But almost every time he saw me, he would talk about what we would do after we got married, where we would go on our honeymoon, how beautiful I was, and how he loved me. Eventually, I just went along with it because I truly didn't know how alert he was, and if he would even remember our conversations anyway. But he sure thought he was charming, and, thankfully, he recovered from having COVID-19 without too many effects of the virus.

## Alfred

Alfred was constantly hungry. He was a resident who had messed up his brain with drugs and now needed long-term care. He reminded me of a 5 year old when he peeked his head out of his room to ask for a cookie. He would take any food left lying around, and if something went missing, we knew where it had gone. When he tested positive for COVID-19, we tried to keep him in his room, but how do you explain to someone who doesn't understand that they can't wander the halls and interact with anyone else, let alone get them to wear a mask on their face. We would do our best to redirect him when he did wander out, and often a snack would do the trick, but he required constant watching. Thankfully, he made a full recovery, as well.

While many of the patients did recover, some were not so fortunate, and it was terribly difficult to see them having trouble breathing and in pain because of their condition. One night, we called a code because one of the residents became unresponsive and was gasping for breath. We waited impatiently while the paramedics came to take him to the hospital. There are some things I will never forget, like the look in his eyes when he had no air to breathe, or the cries of pain from the old woman who would scream and cry out any time someone touched her. We had to clean her and provide care, so hearing her crying in pain was a daily occurrence until the day she passed away.

In May and June, the numbers of positives would continue to rise. Some staff caught the virus and died. The deaths were happening daily at one point. Some of the units lost almost one third of their residents. The nurses and staff had been thrown into this crisis without a choice, and they became overworked and stressed out. There was more work assigned because of the pandemic, and more charting and monitoring. They would talk about what they would do when this was all over. And when they started getting relief workers from all over the country, they were so grateful and thankful for the help.

All the nurses and staff were fighting this thing together against an enemy that was as much mental as it was physical. We stood side by side, locking arms, giving out care and hope the best we could to all of those in our care. It truly became like a family to me. We worked hard, and then even harder to battle what was happening around us in a health care system that was imperfect to begin with. These nurses and caregivers are the real heroes, the ones there before me, and who will still be there after me. Many of us picked up overtime work as well, and some weeks we would work 70+ hours in stressful conditions because the need was so great.

Some days were more bearable than others, but on the difficult days, it felt like I would lose my mind. The PPE (Personal Protective Equipment/wear) was so hot and stifling, and sometimes it felt hard to breath with the N95 mask on and the surgical mask on top of it because we had to reuse the N95 masks for over a week sometimes. There were days when the exhaustion got to me because of the long days on my feet, working without a break at times, and a lack of sleep. What kept me going was the fact that I would see my family again in a few weeks, and my quiet meditations every morning as I started my day by recentering and refocusing my mind. I don't know if I would have made it through without that.

We monitored every resident three times a day for vital signs and any changes in their health condition. We kept a close eye on them as best as we could while they were quarantined in their rooms for months. All the while, being so cautious about wearing our protective gear and changing it out when needed, as well as every point of contact that was made. In fact, one nurse I worked with had a full body hazmat suit that she donned every shift and wore the whole time that she was in the building. We were constantly wiping everything down with cleaning wipes, and most of us were a little paranoid when we left work for home or wherever we were staying. I would change out my shoes when I got to the car and strip out of all my clothes right inside the door of my room. And then I would put those clothes in a separate basket and jump into a hot shower immediately to wash off the day. I washed my hands so many times during the day that my hands became so dry, and the face masks gave me such bad acne that I am still trying to get rid of it.

There were certainly ups and downs on this journey. I became homesick and missed my family terribly. One low point of my time in New Jersey, was the day that the woman who had just celebrated her 103rd birthday became ill with COVID-19. She kept getting sicker and sicker until she quit eating and died a few days later. I shed many tears in those days, but I also became more in touch with my emotions, which was not such a bad thing. This taught me to be a little more vulnerable, and I opened up. This journey was a difficult one for me, and I was very hesitant at first. I had so much doubt and uncertainty. But it has enriched my life in ways I couldn't have even imagined. I have grown personally and mentally, I have learned so much about myself, and I have proved to myself that I can do anything.

Through it all, there were many positive points, like the many Thank You signs and billboards posted around town and the billboards hailing healthcare workers. They even had commercials on TV to say thank you. I received a free airline ticket to New Jersey and back home from United Airlines, I also received a free hotel room from Hilton for the month of May. I got many free cups of coffee and tokens of love from those here in Arizona. I felt so loved and supported and received many cards and gifts in the mail. I found some new friends and met so many great people that I would not have met otherwise. It has been such an empowering discovery and an incredible learning process. I truly made a difference and gave hope to so many people. And for that I will be forever grateful. I appreciate all of the love and support. It meant so much to me during this trying time. And most of all, I appreciate the love and support from my family.

# About Cyndi

CYNDI GRADUATED FROM nursing school almost 9 years ago. She has always had a desire to help others. She is a wife and a mother to three amazing children, and her passion is to care for people. She loves to travel and see new places and try new things; however, her heart is at home with her family. She 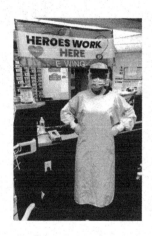 has learned to grow and push herself to new challenges. Moving around a lot and living overseas has given her an appreciation for change and taught her how to be flexible. Above all, she believes in living life to the fullest and taking on life full force. Her desire is to show others how they can change their lives and be healthy. All of this comes with its challenges, but she wouldn't have it any other way.

# Crying is For My Day Off

Kristen Martins

WAKE UP. EAT BREAKFAST. I PUT MY MASK ON AND walk to work in the brisk, early morning sunlight of New Jersey. My shift starts at 07:00. As I walk into the hospital, I am stopped for a forehead temperature scan and asked if I have any flu-like symptoms before proceeding to the ICU. I gather my single N95 mask for the day, a hair net, shoe covers (if available), a plastic gown, and a pair of hospital issued scrubs. I reuse my face shield just like every other day.

I head down two floors to the makeshift ICU. The entrance is blocked off with heavy-duty construction plastic, the hospital's attempt at making the OR and PACU 'negative-pressure.' [COVID can stay airborne for several hours with aerosolization and the negative pressure means particles will flow into the COVID area, not into other surrounding hallways]. This area is filled with people, each crammed side-by-side, with just enough room for a ventilator and a few IV poles between patients.

Reporting is quick and straight to the point. Keep them alive. This place is incredibly noisy. A place of excessive audio and visual stimulation. Constant dinging vents, monitors, IV pumps. Lights flashing on the monitors for low oxygen saturations, low blood pressures, dysrhythmias. Lights flashing on vents for high peak pressures, low minute volumes, low tidal volumes. You have to literally yell to the person next to you because of all the noise, coupled with the muffling that occurs when wearing a respirator and face shield. It is hot. Stressful. And I am rebreathing my exhaled $CO_2$ for the next thirteen hours in these masks. They are so tight that I have bruises behind my ears and wear a Band-Aid on my nose to protect myself from a pressure ulcer.

Supplies in this area are sparse. I run around asking people for saline flushes. Alcohol pads. Linen. We are running out of syringes. Running out of IV fluids. Running out of places to plug in all the electronics that are keeping my patients alive. Needing to prioritize which patient is the sickest and needs priority attention. Stabilize as much as possible and move on to the next. There are between 4-6 critically ill patients per nurse. Each patient has a minimum of three titratable drips and fluids, this means managing a minimum of 12-18 IV pumps, and that is being conservative. We have anesthesiologists and specialized physicians working as attendings. Nurse anesthetists working as attendings. People doing jobs they have never done before this pandemic hit. We must work as a team to keep the patients viable and each other sane. Or mostly sane at least.

I auscultate my patient's lungs. I hear fluid/mucus. They need to be suctioned. We have run out of in-line ETT suction catheters. The only option is sterile suctioning, which requires unhooking the patient from the vent [aka aerosolizing] and putting COVID airborne. But the patient's O2 sats are dropping, their heart rate is increasing, they are visibly in distress. Intervene immediately or risk a respiratory arrest followed by cardiac arrest. Benefit outweighs the risk. Exposed.

I do not beat myself up for not being able to give personal care to any of my patients because keeping them alive is more important. I run my ass off all day and literally have no time to even go to the bathroom myself. I happen to have a few helpers with me on this particular day, which means that my patients can get some much overdue cleaning up. They are with the patient right behind me, giving him a quick turn, wash down, and clean sheets. I hear the alarms start to ring. O2 sats are in the 80s. I give him 100% oxygen and suction down is ETT and in his mouth. They turn him to his left. Flat line. I check the carotid. Nothing. I lower the side rails and get onto the bed, hands on his chest while simultaneously yelling if anyone else feels a pulse?! No pulse. I immediately start CPR. "I NEED HELP! GET THE AED!" I feel his ribs cracking under my palms with each compression. Getting adequate CO2 capnography, meaning compressions are good, at this point. His chest recoil is shit. Doctors are at the bedside. Quickly discussing how long to attempt resuscitation. Epi is given. No pulse. No rhythm. No shock. CPR. Bicarb given. He starts bleeding profusely, spraying bright red blood from his mouth, around the ETT tube, and nose. Code lasts under seven minutes. My first death. This is only 09:20.

This man who had no past medical history, had become so sick that he was requiring daily dialysis. I have said in the past that getting a breathing tube is a death sentence. More accurately, I would say that if a patient gets to the point of needing a dialysis catheter, it is just prolonging 'life'. There has only been one person who wasn't taken to the body trailers after their breathing tube was removed. One.

As soon as one body goes out to the trailers, a new person is admitted from the emergency department, or someone is transferred from the floor who needs ICU care. I admitted three more patients by the end of that shift, giving me the opportunity to care for six patients. One of my admits coded as soon as she got to me. Two codes and two deaths in six hours. I needed to dust myself off and get back at it. I had four other people who needed my best. No time to grieve. Crying is for my days off. When I am alone. When I can process and decompress. My husband and my big sister are my people. I can vent, cuss, cry, yell, scream, feel all the emotions; and they will be there to hold me up, even if it is virtually from 1,200 miles away.

The 19:30 night shift arrives. Fresh faces compared to my sweaty, worn out face. I feel as if I have been hit by a train. Again, the report/handoff is quick and talking about only what is essential. Is anyone teetering on life and death? Is anyone actively trying to die? I wish them luck and leave the unit. I doff my PPE that I put on thirteen hours earlier. I wipe down my face shield for use on my next shift. Noticing that I have been wearing specks of my patient's blood all day. I recognize that my shoulders and chest ache from performing those chest compressions. My mind replays the whole scenario. The pain I experience when removing my mask is a deep ache radiating on all bony prominences of my face and head. I scrub my hands, my arms, my face with soap and water. I put on a simple mask to return to the ICU to change and gather my belongings before walking home.

It is now 20:45. I am walking down the streets, alone. I hear the alarms in my head. They sound like a chorus of emergency vehicle sirens all going off simultaneously. A car occasionally drives by, but it is otherwise silent. It is dark. I feel the brisk cool wind on my face again. I slide my mask down and take a deep, cleansing breath of fresh air. I look up at the stars. My eyes well with tears for those I lost today. As much as I need the rest and the sleep, I know I am needed in that place and I am anxious to go back. I am honored to be able to be a part of something historic and to help save lives each day.

# About Kristen

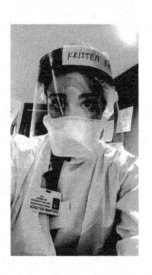

K RISTEN MARTINS, ICU RN. Worked in New Jersey for this COVID contract. Normally/ currently, I work in Saint Paul, Minnesota. Live/from Minneapolis, Minnesota.

# Marching to a Different Beat

Vindy Teja

W HEN IT IS NOT POURING RAIN IN VANCOUVER, MY good friend's sister, Satnam Sekhon, leaves the house at 7:30 each morning and makes her 45-minute march to B.C Cancer, where she works as a dietician. On this particular morning in March 2020, Satnam feels a host of emotions as her mind races with ideas. She needs to focus on something positive to take her mind off her worry.

Being a health care professional for over 30 years, Satnam was feeling the magnitude of what was happening around the world and which was now was impacting her world. As a mother of two health professionals working directly on the frontlines in ICU and Respirology, she sensed the severity and how it would potentially affect her family. Even though she knew this was their passion, just as it was hers, her maternal instincts were making her afraid for them and she was unsure of what to do. She needed to be there for her family. She listened to her inner voice and asked for a leave from work and knew right away it was the right choice.

Her ideas come fast and furious. She makes a mental note of people to enlist and starts calling during her march to work.

And that's when I hear my phone ringing at 7:37 a.m. It wakes me from my deep slumber, and I mean deep. The isolate-at-home recommendations began during my daughter's high school spring break. We quickly fell into the habit of watching movies late into the evening after our dinner routine. The latest was Benjamin Button, a movie we could both agree on because it starred Brad Pitt. Not only did movie time allow us to hit the pause button on our morning school commute, it helped shift our attention away from the ominous and relentless newsfeed.

Satnam sounded perky, impassioned, and full of hope. Even on a bad day, her positive energy is contagious. She possessed a wonderful ability to identify people's talents and motivate them to use them in fun and helpful ways. She had heard my daughter sing at my book launch, so she invited us to join in her efforts to fight COVID-19. Still lacking the effects of java in my bloodstream, I did my best to match her energy. Before long, we had a plan.

"I thought of Kiran's beautiful singing voice and wondered if she'd be willing to record parodies of Backstreet Boys songs to spread the messages about handwashing, physical distancing, and staying home. I can have the lyrics to you in a day or two!" Where does she come up with these ideas?

And that's how early one weekday morning, I got drawn into Satnam's "seyva" assignment. A central teaching in the Sikh households we were both raised in. "Seyva" means "self-giving service." By week's end,

Kiran had recorded two songs that were shared via social media and text group chats. Also, Satnam's son, who worked in ICU, wrote an open impassioned letter about how imperative it was to heed public health safety messages. It was widely circulated. The message was having an impact!

I suggested to Satnam that her sons do a social media post holding signs imploring the public to protect themselves and healthcare workers by washing their hands, physical distancing, and staying home. I had seen similar hard-hitting posts on social media.

"Let's do it," read her reply. Twenty seconds later, another text, "Can you have signs translated? Punjabi, Mandarin, French, etc.?"

I enlisted my retired Auntie Manjit's help to do the Punjabi translation because she volunteered as a translator. Kiran studies Spanish and did those signs. Her friend Dylan emailed the French translations fifteen minutes after I asked him.

Who did I know who could write other languages relevant to Vancouver's diverse community? I took a chance and emailed Josephine, a family lawyer and journalism student I hadn't even met but who interviewed me recently in my capacity as a Divorce Coach about the impact of COVID-19 on separated and divorced couples. To my delight, she did the signs in formal and informal Chinese in less than an hour!

I was so impressed with *everyone's* willingness to help. All of them were everyday heroes. If it hadn't been for the glue, a.k.a. Satnam, holding everyone and everything together, the domino effect wouldn't have been the same.

When Satnam and her team invited me to join them regularly during COVID-19, I learned something new about her. She and my friend had started a community organization over twenty years earlier called SEYVA. The group not only embodied the spirit of the word "seyva", it was also an acronym highlighting the power of pairing a fun learning environment with the desire to help others: Socializing and Educating Youth through Volunteer Activities. The group raised money to send children with disabilities to camp, engaged with senior homes, helped terminally ill children, and did shore clean-up and clothing drives. I was struck by what this small group of dedicated volunteers had accomplished.

At the start of the COVID-19 crisis, SEYVA adapted and became SEYVA at HOME. Satnam regrouped alumni and included new members to address the community's immediate needs. She recognized that the food banks would be a much-needed resource for months to come.

In the spirit of Vaisakhi, a parade commemorating the birth of Sikhism and celebration with food, SEYVA thought to contribute in a slightly different way. They used their platform to do a virtual Vaisakhi Food Drive to raise funds for the Greater Vancouver Food Bank. If people couldn't attend Vaisakhi in 2020, then SEYVA would take it where it was needed! In a few short weeks, with community support, we raised close to $25,000, which allowed the Food Bank to purchase almost $75,000 worth of food for their clients.

Thank you, Satnam, for waking me up from my deep slumber at 7:37 in the morning during your march to work. It allowed me to march to the beat of an important drum...raising community safety awareness and helping those most affected by COVID-19.

## About Vindy

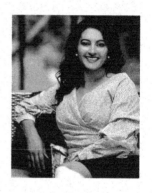

V INDY TEJA IS A TEDx
Speaker, Professional Life
& Divorce Coach, and Author.
She's a graduate of UBC and
Western Law School. Following
her call to the bar, Vindy dis-
covered her coaching passion as
Career Development Director at
Western Law School. Along with many joys and suc-
cesses, she's dealt with serious setbacks and challenges,
not to mention pesky self-doubts. The result? Her book
*YOLO: Essential Life Hacks for Happiness*, a practi-
cal and meaningful dive into deconstructing happiness,
and an anthology in which she is co-author: *Passed
Down From Mom: A Collection of Inspiring Stories
About Moms & Motherhood*. www.vindyteja.com

# About Satnam

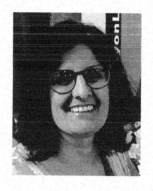

S ATNAM WROTE A COOKBOOK (she's a dietician after all) so I pulled the following biography and added the cookbook credentials. Use the details you think would work as I know it has to be a certain length for the anthology.

Satnam Sekhon is a Registered Dietician, UBC Clinical Instructor with the Faculty of Land and Food Systems, and author of cookbook "Dhaal-icious: Indian Meals From My Kitchen To Yours". She has dedicated her professional career in cancer care for over 30 years while actively volunteering at the grassroots community level with provincial and national organizations.

Satnam co-founded SEYVA (Socializing and Educating Youth through Volunteer Activities), helping to fundraise for local charities. Satnam and her husband Harman enjoy opening their home to family, friends and sometimes complete strangers to share a hearty, home-cooked meal.

# Some Heroes Wear Scrubs

## Archana Shrestha

ROM THE VERY FIRST TIME I WORKED IN THE EMER-
gency room (ER) as a medical student at an inner-city
Chicago hospital, I knew the Emergency Department
was the place where everyday heroes roamed. The doctors, the nurses, the paramedics all had that swagger,
confidence and calm even under extreme pressure,
that only emergency professionals and first responders
can have. They were like Greek gods and goddesses to
me. They had what it takes to save lives, save limbs and
even deliver babies. Gun shots, overdoses, and shock-
ing patients out of fatal arrhythmias. One fire put out
after the next. They have gone to the edge of life and
death and been able to bring back many, but not all.
There are times when no effort, not even the heroic efforts of the men and women who work in the ER, can
save a person. In those moments, these heroes had
grace and knew exactly how to approach talking to the
loved ones of the deceased. And after having that con-
versation, they knew how to compose themselves and
go on with their shifts to see the next patient whose
emergency needed to be addressed.

The ER was an exciting place for a bright-eyed medical student eager to make a difference. I was enamored
by the aura of these everyday heroes of the ER. This
was medicine on the frontlines. The adrenaline rush
was intoxicating, and it was where my dream of being
an everyday hero was born.

Fast forward nearly two decades later. I have been working in the ER as a doctor for 15 years. Now, as an emergency physician in the middle of a global pandemic, I have lost count of just how many COVID 19 patients I have taken care of in the emergency room. I recall my first COVID patient: an elderly woman in her 70s. Her daughter, who was in her 40s, had just been placed on a ventilator in our ER after being brought in by ambulance with severe trouble breathing. My patient, though elderly with a few chronic medical problems including emphysema and congestive heart failure, luckily didn't look so sick when she came into the hospital. This was despite the fact that she lived in the same home with her ill daughter and the fact that they had also been sharing an inhaler and unintentionally spreading Coronavirus to one another. My patient's husband was also in the ER in the room next to her. And it turned out that their granddaughter, the daughter of the 40 something year old, was the first to catch the Coronavirus. What we were seeing was a family cluster of cases. It was the beginning of the Coronavirus storm that we emergency physicians had been bracing for in our community.

In medical school we never had a class on what to do in a pandemic. In an era of vaccines which have stamped out measles and smallpox worldwide, the thought of a global pandemic killing hundreds of thousands of people in this day and age seemed unfathomable. Even as the news reports of Coronavirus spreading through China came to light, many in the medical community here in the United States didn't expect it to spread so widely here.

But the spring of 2020 brought with it not only flowers blooming and baby chicks hatching, but also Coronavirus to our shores. My state of Illinois shut down schools in mid-March and, a week later, the entire state was on a stay-at-home-order. We, emergency physicians, and the rest of the ER and hospital staff were still needed on the frontlines. So, as nearly my entire neighborhood and extended family got to stay safe at home, I went off to the ER to serve my community, leaving my husband and our two school-aged children at home.

My anxiety rose especially as I listened to news reports of nationwide shortages of personal protective equipment (PPE) and of States outbidding one another to secure more. We all worried about shortages of PPE in our own ER and some days the charge nurses would tell me we were running low. Luckily, I was able to purchase some of my own and have some shipped in from relatives living internationally. This allowed me to be protected and safer while caring for patients with Coronavirus. But no matter how careful I was, I knew I was still at risk for catching Coronavirus from work just as one of my physician colleagues and numerous nurses had working in the same ER as me. All of us were at high risk of catching COVID-19, but the definition of courage is feeling the fear and continuing to do it anyway. And so it was that all of us in the ER—doctors, nurses, techs, phlebotomists, respiratory therapists, house keepers, and security guards—courageously went into work to care for all of our patients including those with COVID. After all, the ER never ever closes, and we truly are the safety net for our communities.

And while I have been a calm, collected, and even-keeled emergency room physician for the 15 years that I have worked in the ER, for the first time in my life I began to feel anxiety. Will I get sick myself? Will I accidentally infect my children, husband or elderly parents? What if both my husband and I catch Coronavirus, who will look after the kids?

I take vitamins and herbal remedies and started prioritizing my sleep more in order to keep my immune system strong in case I do catch it. I talk to counselors and life coaches to manage my anxiety about being on the frontlines of COVID 19. I do whatever it takes to be able to show up to my shift for my patients and my community.

I wake up each morning of my shift and give myself a pep talk. *"You know how to protect yourself in the ER,"* I tell myself. "You are young and healthy and strong." The affirmations help me to get in the right frame of mind to go to work.

At work, I park my car in the parking lot and grab my big bag of personal PPE from my trunk. First, I don my freshly washed white coat which bears my name and credentials, then I put on my surgical mask because without a mask we cannot enter the hospital. I enter the employee entrance and my temperature is checked. I am asked a series of questions to screen if I have any COVID 19 symptoms. I badge into the ER and the double doors sweep open to a sea of fellow ER staff who are wearing bonnets, blue scrubs and face masks. Even though I have worked at this same hospital for over a decade, under the face masks it's hard to tell who is who anymore. Before sitting down at my computer workstation in the ER, I wipe down the entire area with a germicidal wipe. We have to be cautious now, more than ever before, to not inadvertently catch the virus from asymptomatic staff members. I put on a surgical bonnet to cover my long hair and shoe covers to prevent spreading germs from my footwear. As I log into the computer and the tracking board, I see my next patient is from a nursing home that has sadly had an outbreak of COVID 19. I put on my N95 mask for the day and, though it is suffocating, I wear it for nearly all of my 10-hour shift. I also put on my safety goggles to protect my eyes as aerosolized Coronavirus can also enter humans through the eyes. I walk into the room to see the patient, and I already know based on his symptoms that he is going to come back positive for the virus. Even inside the exam room I keep a distance of 6 feet. It's difficult for us to hear and understand one another as we are both wearing masks, but we push through communicating the crucial information. It's hard to establish rapport with a patient who cannot see your full facial expressions. I know all the PPE we must wear to protect ourselves makes the whole experience scarier for patients. I step closer for a few minutes to examine the patient then step back towards the door telling him I will let him know his results once they are all back. His results come back confirming my suspicion that he does indeed have COVID 19. Due to his oxygen levels also running low, I tell him we will keep him in the hospital to monitor him. Even though he doesn't have severe COVID symptoms at this time, in my mind I say a prayer for him knowing that things could go the way they did for my very first Corona patient, the woman in her 70s, who unfortunately ended up dying alone in the hospital with only the nurses by her side. When someone with COVID 19 is about to die, not even family members are allowed to say good-bye in person. They must say their final "I love you" over the phone or by video.

The shift goes on, usually with me caring for numerous patients with COVID. Finally, it is time for me to go home and my decontamination routine commences with wiping down all my equipment and my cell phone so I don't take any germs home with me. As soon as I get outdoors into the fresh air, I take a big deep breath filling my lungs with gratitude for how great it feels to breathe without a mask on.

When I arrive home, I leave my work shoes in the garage and head straight down to the basement to what I now call my "COVID shower." I have a special hamper for the used scrubs and white coat. I hop in for a long hot shower and always wash my hair as COVID has been known even to stick to hair. My long tresses have now become frizzy from over-washing. I dare not embrace my husband and kids until this ritual is complete. But when I come back upstairs after decontaminating, I'm greeted with big bear hugs. I have missed my family and they have missed me. Each day when I go to work, they along with my extended family are at home worrying about their mamma and wife.

Finally, as the day ends, I lay my head down on my pillow. And even though I'm physically exhausted, worry keeps me awake. Being an everyday hero is hard. It was hard before the pandemic, and it is even harder now that I worry for my own safety in the ER and that I might bring illness home to my family. I ponder that "Maybe I don't want to be a hero any longer." Have I done enough to serve my community? Have I saved enough lives in the 15 years I have worked in the ER both day and night? Have I worked enough weekends and holidays away from my husband and children?

I just want to be able to watch my kids grow up to become adults. I want to grow old with my husband. And one day I'd like to become a grandma too. Is that too much to ask? Isn't my duty as mother and wife more important than my career as a physician? Must heroes sacrifice themselves for others forever? Or does there come a time when even heroes too have done enough?

I wake up the next day, eyes groggy from a night spent worrying, and head to work to care for patients in the ER. But in the back of my mind, as I don all my PPE about to enter the room of confirmed COVID positive patient, I hear my intuition whispering that there's got to be another way. I search my mind for ways I might serve patients while also protecting my family and caring for my children who are home doing remote e-learning for the foreseeable future. Could there be another way for me to practice medicine beyond the walls of the ER?

Then I recall how for many years I had been thinking of getting started in telemedicine and seeing patients virtually. I hear from colleagues practicing telemedicine of the large uptick in patients seeking virtual care and the long wait times to be seen over telemedicine as so many patients don't want to go into a hospital or clinic for fear of catching Coronavirus.

I decide to give telemedicine a try and after seeing my first few patients virtually, I realize I absolutely love telemedicine and so do the patients. They love the convenience of getting to see a doctor from the comfort of their homes and at any time they need help. I also love how efficient telemedicine is and how in one hour, I'm able to help so many more people virtually than I am in person in the ER. My telemedicine patients are so incredibly grateful for what I do for them from the safety of their own home. "This is amazing and you're a God send!" one patient says. "You're my savior!" says another.

I realize now that in this day and age, an everyday healthcare hero can show up in different ways, sometimes standing next to you in the ER and other times over a screen in your home. But regardless of whether in-person or virtually the care I provide is the same - compassionate, caring and always putting the patient first. And no matter if I'm working in the ER or virtually from home, when I'm caring for patients, I always put on my scrubs and white coat because when I do I immediately transform myself into someone who is ready to help and be an everyday hero.

# About Archana

D R. ARCHANA SHRESTHA IS an emergency physician, life coach, bestselling author, speaker and entrepreneur. She is the co-founder of Women in White Coats and the founder and chief wellness officer at Mighty Mom, MD.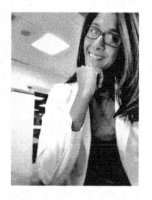

In addition to being a board-certified emergency medicine physician, Archana is also an Assistant Professor of Emergency Medicine in the Department of Clinical Sciences at Rosalind Franklin University of Medicine and Science. She obtained her undergraduate and medical degrees from the University of Illinois at Chicago and completed emergency medicine residency at George Washington University. As a medical student, she was awarded a prestigious Fulbright Fellowship for the study of medical anthropology in Ecuador.

Archana also earned a Masters in Journalism from the University of Illinois at Champaign-Urbana. Passionate about medical journalism, she interned at the ABC News Medical Unit in Boston. In addition to serving as co-editor-in-chief of the Women in White Coats blog, to which she is a regular contributor, her writing has been published by ABC News, the Chicago Sun Times, KevinMD and Doximity. She is also the co-author of the bestselling book series, "The Chronicles of Women in White Coats."

Archana was honored with the Women in Medicine Summit #SheforShe Honorable Mention Award in 2020 for her work supporting and advocating for women physicians. She was also honored as one of the 2018 Top 20 Global Women of Excellence by U.S. Congressman Danny K. Davis in recognition of her achievements not only in medicine and journalism but also as a life coach and entrepreneur who empowers busy working mothers to achieve holistic wellness through her healthy living lifestyle blog called MightyMomMD.com. As a working mom of two herself, Archana's mission is to uplift and empower working women, in particular women in healthcare.

# First day,
# to be essential
# or not essential?

Brigit Anderson

M Y WORK HAS ALWAYS CHALLENGED AND REWARDED me in amazing ways. I've felt blessed to do this work as an occupational therapist for the past 20 years, with experience in skilled nursing facilities, rehabilitation, inpatient acute care, outpatient lymphedema, to inpatient intensive care, trauma and critical care.

And then 2020 came. COVID-19 (COVID) hit.

My work is inconceivable. Working with COVID patients is the hardest thing I've ever done. My patients were in the ICU and the sickest people I've ever seen in my 20 years of working in the field.

When COVID first popped up, my work was impacted by making all therapy non-essential for all COVID patients. I did what I could to support my friends and colleagues working with COVID patients. I offered my spare bedroom,and laundry for those whose family was at high risk plus listened and loved on people I've known for years to help them move from day to day.

Weeks into the virus, my life went from normal to war zone.

Walking into the hospital changed almost overnight. For years, I could anticipate the energy of a hospital.

Hustle and bustle.

Lots of family and friends pouring over their loved ones with care.

All of that changed when I walked into the hospital once COVID came. It was eerie. It was a ghost town. No noise on some floors. I imagine it had the same deafening silence as a village or town does after an attack of some kind.

The COVID Floors were the exact opposite. Alarms going off, IV's constantly beeping, people everywhere, PPE. Gear lined up outside every room. People walking the halls with respirators, N95 masks, face shields, constantly dressing or undressing PPE depending if they were going in or coming out of a room and washing hands over and over again.

Going up to the ICU after weeks of "non-essential" status was unlike anything I've seen in a hospital, yet as part of its daily life. It took a committee of high-level staff to decide my job as an occupational therapist was essential.

I remember mentioning to my director at the very beginning of COVID that I knew in my bones that my job, and that of other therapists around the country, was essential. That was never an issue. The issue was that nobody knew how these patients would respond. Whether they would live? And if they did, how they would live. Through all these "ifs," when would my job and that of others like me be brought into the equation.

I found the answer to these questions a little more than a month after COVID hit. Therapy was considered essential.

When therapists were finally assigned COVID patients, it felt a lot like it does when I missed an important meeting. Or walked into a party when everyone else left. Or that feeling that happens when everyone else knows an inside joke.

From the start, I was playing catch up. It was maddening. And since this was such a new experience, no one knew what to do or when to get therapy involved; there was no end in sight. I was always behind.

But so was every other healthcare professional working around the world.

As a therapist, I wasn't brought in until the COVID patients had progressed to a certain point and looked as though he/she was heading in the right direction.

I knew COVID patients would be profoundly weak. Many of them had been near death. Most of them had required a ventilator and laid in bed for weeks. They had been unable to move a limb even by a centimeter off the bed. Many had experienced so many complications. And yet, they were now alive and moving toward recovery!

I braced myself mentally for that first day, making sure I was as emotionally ready as I possibly could be. But really, nobody is ever prepared for something like that.

Putting on full COVID gear is quite an experience. I stripped down from the scrubs I had on into a new pair of scrubs. I put on my shoe covers, hair cover, an N95 mask, and a face shield. Over all of that, is a plastic gown cover and finally double gloves, just in case a glove rips or a change is needed.

As I approach the room, I realize this is the first COVID patient being treated by therapy services in our ICU. Finally, after some time therapy is considered "essential."

I'm grateful to be able to play a part in the treatment of these patients. In my opinion, therapy is always essential in overall wellbeing and care. So, I think to myself, all I can do is what I have always done. I start at the beginning and progress the patient as is appropriate.

I take a deep breath and, along with my counterpart physical therapist, we prepare to enter the room. I peek through the glass doors. The patient's bed is turned backwards. All I see is the back of the patient's head. That's different. The sliding doors are shut with spaghetti-like IV lines snaking over the bed through the room and reaching the door frame where it is anchored there by using foley catheters anchors. Nurses rearranged the room to anchor the IV to the door frame. Ingenious! Nurses are amazing!

Why is the patient's room set up this way? This way, medications can be given without entering the room which saves PPE! All the lines lead to the IV pumps outside the room, with the vent control panel anchored outside the room on the supply cart, usually in the room.

My heart starts beating with anticipation. We are getting him upright and out of bed for the first time! Normally, entering and exiting a room is possible without too much difficulty, but with "full COVID contact precautions," it's not so easy!

I have to first ask myself what is already in the room, what is needed and what I may need once I'm in there. To say the least, this is incredibly intense! I've worked in this ICU for years and it doesn't look anything close to what it usually looks like. I don't know where anything is and I put all of that out of my head, take a deep breath and get to work.

Working with a patient with profound body wasting is a challenge to say the least. He has no movement, is vent dependent, weak, fatigued, covered in wounds from the rotoprone bed (bed that allows patients to be turned upside down to breathe easier) and has poor cognition.

My first COVID patient is young. He's in his early 30s. I can see him smiling at me through the vent tubing. He actually calms my nerves a little bit. Even though his smile is weak, he is awake with a bit of attention. He seems happy to see people regardless of the fact that we may look like aliens to him. He doesn't know the date, where he is, and is confused yet following commands with lots of extra time.

I am so surprised he is so young. The reports I had read about COVID up to that point were that the virus hit the elderly the hardest. But this patient is in his early 30s, even though he is overweight and pre-diabetic.

I run through the list of questions I ask every patient and he can answer half of them with a simple yes or no.

I'm ready to get to work and yet, my job is not like normal. There are new challenges.

I look around the room and the bed and patient and ask myself, "How am I supposed to move him when critical lines can't be moved?"

I have space that is only two feet by two feet. It's not nearly enough space to move a patient. All lines connected to him are critical and can't be moved. He's ventilated, which is critical and super important so that can't be moved!

Minutes go by. I examine and think about every move I could make and the repercussions it could have on my patient.

If I move him like that, this line could disconnect.

If I move him like this, that line could disconnect.

Finally, after some time, I roll him, which takes more effort than anticipated. With all my gear on, and the ventilator, it takes maximum effort to assist him to the edge of the bed. To help him maintain a seated position during our therapy session is even harder. My whole body shakes. I'm using every muscle I didn't know I had, combined with an overdrive of adrenaline.

It's difficult to breathe through the mask. I'm at the point of exhaustion due to the massive amount of effort required to sustain another human being in an upright position for so long while attempting to breathe in an N95 mask.

Sweat drips down my back.

I'm soaked actually. And this is just the first patient. I have three more to go.

Our initial therapy session is called "drag and sit." We are just going to sit on the edge of the bed and brush his teeth with a tube down his throat.

Who knew a simple task could be so awesome? Brushing my teeth is something I've never taken for granted since that day. It's the first time that movement other than a typical range of motion is possible!

He tolerates about 10 minutes, requiring two people to assist with sitting up on the edge of the bed, participating in all activity and laying back down and for repositioning. Sweat pours out from every pore. I'm drenched. I can barely see due to the condensation from heavy breathing and start to hyperventilate.

There's this wave of anxiety that washes over me.

What if I pass out? I think.

What if I can't do this for him, I think pull it together man!

Focus. You can do this.

It's almost over.

Ok.

Done.

Now the backward procedure. I have to remove my gown and gloves without touching the outside of the gown or glove. I have to wash my hands, remove my mask, glasses, and shield and then wash both.

It's all worth it though. Seeing a person start the momentous journey to recovery gets me excited and I take a deep breath to get ready to do it all over again.

I see three more COVID patients that day, after seeing regular patients in the morning.

And each patient is harder than the last one. My body is wrecked with exertion due to having all my COVID gear on. With the new physical demands needed to do my job, the morale on the ICU floor is different. There is overwhelm, and new hyper vigilance in the air ...and one perk, music is allowed to reduce stress. My nerves and the feeling of being useless are gone and replaced with passion and drive again.

It's the end of the first day of working with COVID patients and I'm finally at my final step of the protection routine.

I wash my hands and gear.

I remove my hair cover and shoe coverings.

I wash my hands again.

I change back into my regular work clothes.

I go home after that first day with a heat rash, serious facial marks from the mask, soaking wet, exhausted with the start of a piercing headache.

The next day came too soon and, without thinking, I moved all my pain and aches aside and got in the mindset necessary to do this work.

Working in the ICU with COVID patients busts open a new frontier. I wonder each day what else I'm in for and how it will look.

How can I make this doable? The frailty of these patients is overwhelming.

Each patient is different, a different size, shape, age, population and all the same to me. Working with them is crazy hard.

Even though helping people is what I love and, giving people the possibility of their lives back brings a smile to my heart and makes it well worth the effort, the next day comes and my body is struggling. I can't ignore the pain. I'm nauseated, with a migraine-like headache all day from what can only be attributed to lack of oxygen during a massive physical exertion.

The number of COVID patients has drastically dropped over the last few months and we are finally going back to the initial set up. We have one unit of COVID in the ICU and a few on the floors.

When COVID first hit, I did self-isolate from my family and friends, which was tough considering how drastic my career demands amplified and I really needed a support outlet. My parents would drive by on my lunch break and I would talk to them through their car window from six-feet away.

Things are slowly returning to normal. Visitors are coming back to the hospital for a few hours daily and elective surgery is up and running again. We are on an honor system to "self-screen" ourselves for COVID.

I never thought I'd see anything like that in my lifetime.

I hope I never do again.

# About Brigit

B RIGIT ANDERSON IS FROM THE San Francisco bay area via Colorado. She is an Occupational therapist, educated at Colorado State University graduating in 2001, currently licensed and working in Arizona at a level one trauma, stroke center in Scottsdale, AZ. She specializes in ICU trauma, strokes, and critical care patients. She is a certified lymphedema therapist (CLT) 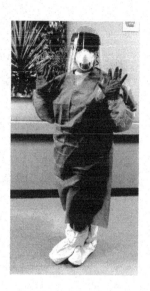 in the Casley-Smith method. Her passion for patient advocacy drives her to provide the best care for each individual patient's needs every day. During her daily activities, she was presented with a patient that allowed her to develop the S.A.C (support and compress) protocol for scrotal edema, and the SuperUNIfit for genital edema male or female. She is single, a proud auntie of 5 amazing nieces and nephews and smiles when they call her auntie BAE 'best auntie ever". She is an avid traveler, living abroad twice, visiting most of Europe, China, New Zealand and Australia. Because of her passion for personal development she's attended several advanced workshops on communication and leadership and is currently involved in a Mastermind group focusing on supporting her local community, and fellow members by reaching for excellence in all areas of life. She adores reading Brene Brown and Joe Dispenza books focusing on becoming the best version of herself. When taking a break from sharing about the SAC protocol and the SuperUNIfit you'll find her spending time, supporting and laughing with friends and family or participating in hot yoga, cycling or on a hike.

# I Made a Difference to that One

## Candy Leigh

S OMETIMES, YOUR FRIEND SUDDENLY BECOMES YOUR hero.

When I met Stacy, we were both fresh meat (rookie skaters) for the Brewcity Bruisers, the roller derby team in Milwaukee, Wisconsin. There were a lot of us trying out that year, so I didn't get to know her well. What I did learn about Stacy (aka House of Pain) was that she was strong on the track: her hips could knock you down and her killer stares could knock you out. You see, derby is both physical and mental, and "Pain" could play the game. Pain and I were drafted to different teams and because of that spent most of our derby time with different skaters. Yet we were part of the same rookie class in the same league, and that bonded us as sisters for life, no matter where life's journeys take us.

This year, when COVID hit, the world was jolted into a state of "in between" existence. Time has now been forever marked as this "dash" that exists only to connect our pre-COVID and post-COVID world. In previous national and international crises, we've been able to collectively rely on the intelligence and expertise of leaders to help us understand and organize and successfully make it through to the other side of the "dash." This time, at the epicenter of the US crisis and in an absence of national unifying leadership, New York's Governor Cuomo became the voice of reason and leadership to move his state and the nation from fear of the virus into a new normal state of existence. During the height of the pandemic, NYC encountered a shortage of nurses. They were burned out, some sick, and some dying, all due to the overwhelming cases and complications of COVID-19. Governor Cuomo initiated a call to bring in healthcare workers to help fill the void, as a result, and Stacy answered that call.

As a roller girl, Pain is tough as nails, but that's nothing compared to Nurse Stacy Ellis. Stacy has been nursing for 10 years. While she spent her early years working in hospitals, she eventually transferred to home health care, which offered more flexibility to balance her work schedule while caring for her 8-year-old daughter. During the months leading up to COVID, she had been exploring travel nursing options, but was worried about whether she had enough experience to pursue that as a career. While she craved stability and routine, she was also hungry to see new places and have new experiences. After several conversations and much soul searching, Stacy decided to make the leap and take a 13-week contract to work in Alabama. Just before she signed on, a fellow nurse mentioned the significant shortage of healthcare workers in New York City, and that some agencies were deploying nurses within 24 hours.

Amid a massive international health pandemic, with no clear facts or unifying message, plan or even an idea of how this crisis would end, Stacy was moved to help NYC, to go where she was needed. She made an initial exploratory call to a local agency on Wednesday afternoon, and she deployed to NYC on Friday morning.

Stacy committed to a rotation of 14-21 days, knowing she would work up to 84-hours per week. She understood the potential danger to her personal health, and she took to heart the time she would be away from her daughter, which would include 2 weeks in quarantine upon her return home. That was, of course, assuming she would not get sick with the virus and would be physically able to return home. After considering all the risks, Nurse Stacy Ellis decided to selflessly answer the call that had landed on her heart. While many ran in the other direction, called the virus "a hoax," or ridiculed others for their belief in science, Stacy walked directly into the fire so that she could offer care and compassion to those who needed her the most.

Nurse Stacy Ellis, House of Pain, stayed in NYC not 2 weeks, not 3, but a total of 50 days, or 7 full work weeks, serving in a NYC hospital on the front lines of the COVID crisis.

She recalls the day she left her home in Texas and arrived in New York:

*"I was the strangest combination of excited, scared and nervous. The airport was a dead*

zone. *Ticket agents made comments about me not being able to come back home. They said I was on the last flight to JFK and that JFK, itself, might be shut down. I watched my suitcase roll down the belt. I had a lump in my throat. I thought about just going back home. There was so much unknown, and this was so far out of my comfort zone. I am a planner, and I had literally no idea what I was walking into. My staffing agency basically said: "Show up here at this time and we will find a job for you." I didn't have any other information. When I got to security, I fumbled my way through TSA. I knew I had to do things like take off my shoes and remove electronics from bags, but I couldn't even figure out which line to walk through.*

*When I boarded the plane, it was all but empty. There were 7 passengers and 3 flight attendants. It was quiet and eerie. I was flying into a place that is known as one of the busiest cities in the world, and basically no one wanted to travel there. When I landed in NYC the reality of the pandemic started to sink in. Everyone was wearing masks, and the federal government hadn't even suggested it yet. I took a hired car from the airport to the hotel, and it was a ghost town. The streets were completely empty, and it was 1:00 p.m. on a Friday. The driver said that normally there would be bumper to bumper traffic, even in the middle of the night. It felt like a scene from "I am Legend." I tried to quiet my mind, but my brain kept swirling with the unknowns of what would come in the next hours and days. I tried to think about nursing skills to push back my fears. I focused on the mandatory quarantine I would have to do when I arrived home. I planned who would drop off tacos and beer on my doorstep. I was scared and stressed. I cried a little bit, but then let that go. The time for that had passed. It was go time."*

Upon her arrival, Stacy settled into her hotel room and her new routine. Nearly every morning for 7 weeks, Stacy got on a cold, quiet bus at 5:40 a.m. with other hero nurses, from around the country, who had answered the call to help our fellow Americans in NYC. At 6:30 a.m. Stacy and the team that would grow to become her family, would arrive at the hospital, receive their orders, and get to work. At 7:30 p.m., they would get back on the bus for the hour-long ride back to their hotel, oftentimes ordering food during the drive if the agency hadn't provided dinner for that day. Once at the hotel, the nurses had to shower and change clothes before picking up any packages from the mail-room. Errands to the drug store or post office were done during the evening. After working 13-hour shifts, getting some food, and taking care of daily tasks, Stacy typically settled into bed at about 11:00 p.m., then she woke up when her alarm went off and went through the same routine all over again.

During her first week in New York, Stacy met Jessica. Jessica had been assigned to the emergency room (ER) just a few days after Stacy's arrival. Neither of them routinely worked in the ER, so it was new ter-ritory for them. On Jessica's first day, Stacy saw she was overwhelmed and unsure of what to do or how to help. "That must have been my face a few days ago," she thought. Without hesitation, Stacy took Jessica under her wings, showing her what was most helpful and what needed to be done. The two of them instant-ly bonded. They tried to take lunch breaks together (when they got them) and days off together. They got groceries and went to the post office together. They checked in with each other all day every day, even when they weren't working in the same area. Jessica and Stacy became each other's *person*. They counted on each other and helped carry each other through the highs and lows of every day, every week...the entire experience.

During those early days, Americans from around the country watched what was happening in New York in a state of disbelief. Mainstream messaging often referred to COVID as a hoax, and leaders claimed it was "under control" and would just "go away." As we know now, that wasn't the case. COVID silently and invisibly marched into people's bodies, stealing their breath and sometimes their lives. In Stacy's first 3 weeks on deployment, she saw countless patients, and countless deaths.

*"What hit me the hardest was the fast progression of COVID. I can't tell you how many patients I saw walk into the ER, talking and alert, and the next day their symptoms had progressed so badly that they needed to be intubated. By the third day those patients were often close to dying or had already died! There aren't words for the helplessness we experienced. I worked in acute ER, where patients needed high-flow oxygen or were already intubated. I will never forget the look on the faces of patients who were transferred into my area. They saw the men and women already in this area, intubated, sedated;*

*they saw the codes every few hours, and they were fully aware that they could easily be next. That realization, that expression of desperation...that is a look of panic and hopelessness and fear that I will never forget. In those moments of uncertainty, I held my patients' hands and reassured them that we were giving them the best care we possibly could. I wanted to calm their anxiety and give them hope, but we all knew that some people weren't going to get better. More times than I would like to remember, I left my shift saying goodbye to healthy patients, only to return in the morning to find them intubated and sedated because their lungs just couldn't fight the virus. Sometimes the hands I held the day before were already lifeless. It was absolutely devastating."*

Even though there was extreme devastation, some patients defeated the virus and eventually left the hospital. They survived. Amid all the uncertainty, anxiety and fear, the survivors were the rays of light, the hope that the family of nurses held onto.

*"We had one man walk into the hospital alert and, for all intents and purposes, "normal."*

*He had typical symptoms for COVID-19 (fever, shortness of breath, cough), and he tested positive. His case seemed mild, but within a few days he deteriorated so much that he became confused and unresponsive. We determined that the man had a stroke, likely related to COVID. Now he was non-verbal, unable to follow simple commands, unable to walk and unable to feed and care for himself.*

*On the first day I took care of him, he only spoke incomprehensible mumbles. He couldn't tell me his name, and he couldn't answer any of my simple questions appropriately. As a nurse, I always assess my patient's level of consciousness, their alertness and orientation. Subtle changes help me recognize a change in condition, whether for better or worse. Because family members know their loved ones better than I do, I usually ask them to help me assess a patient's behaviors. Unfortunately, with COVID, there are no family members at the bedside. Patients are left alone. It adds a layer of uncertainty for all of us. Everything is up to the nurse. It's up to me.*

*Every time I was in this patient's room, I assessed him, hoping for signs of improvement. I asked questions and talked to him, observing how he responded to me. He would squeeze my hand, sometimes so hard it hurt. I would tell him he was hurting me and to let go just a little, and he did. I would still hold his hand and talk to him. I knew he was trying to communicate, that he had something he wanted to say. With each passing day, I noticed he was more alert, making more eye contact, watching my every move, grabbing my hand on command. I just kept talking to him and reassuring him that he would be alright. My heart broke every time I looked in his eyes because I knew he had something to say; his words were trapped inside a body that was not responding to his mind.*

*One day when my shift was about to end, I made one last visit to his room to check on him. When I walked in, he made direct eye contact with me and seemed more alert than usual, but, still, no words. I talked to him and did my best to make sure he was comfortable. He kept following me with those eyes. Those eyes. I looked directly at him. I squeezed his* hand. I smiled and told him I would see him tomorrow. I turned to walk out the door, and just before I left his room, he said out loud, plain as day, "Can I call my wife?" I stopped dead in my tracks. I was completely shocked. I whipped around: "WHAT!?" My patient looked directly at me and said it again, "Can I call my wife?" I was amazed. "YES! What is your wife's name?" He told me her name, then he told me her phone number. His speech was still garbled from the stroke, so I ran to my computer to confirm the number. I quickly wrote it down, shaking and hurrying because I had no idea how long he would be alert and talkative. I ran back to his room and picked up his phone. The battery was just about dead, so I hopped over IV poles and feeding tubes and cords and all kinds of obstacles to get the charger plugged into the wall. Once I finally got it plugged in, I dialed the number. It rang once and his wife answered. The words spilled quickly out of my mouth, "This is your husband's nurse, and he wants to talk to you." I handed him the phone.

The memory of that moment and the echo of those words will never leave my heart or

*mind. Experiencing that moment of awaken-
ing and communication was one of the most
profound moments of my life. She cried. He
cried. I cried. My patient, who had been alone
in the hospital and unresponsive for 2 weeks,
talked to his wife and his son, who had been
alone and afraid for 2 weeks, simply hoping that he would live and that they would
hear each other's voices again. I stood back
against the wall and silently sobbed, trying
not to ruin the one N95 mask that had been
rationed to me for that week. I listened as he
tried to speak clearly and answer their questions. This man, in his mid-50s, who couldn't
stand and couldn't take care of himself, re-
peatedly reassured his wife and son that he
was okay. He told them not to worry about
him. He used all the strength he could mus-
ter to ask how THEY were. He asked about
his son's school. He reminded his son to take
care of his mom, since he couldn't be there
to take care of her himself. He told them he
loved them and that he would be alright.*

*Over the next few days, my patient's health
continued to improve, and he eventually
transferred to a rehab facility to regain the*

*skills needed to go home. I often wonder and can only hope that he is home now, home with his wife and his son.*

*To my last day, I will be forever thankful and call myself lucky that I was the person in the room that day when, after days of not speaking at all, he was finally able to say, "Can I call my wife?"*

After 50 days of taking care of patients who were fighting an invasive and elusive virus, Stacy was ready to leave New York and return home. She was excited to be with her daughter. She was homesick. It was time. When they asked if she would come back, she laughed nervously and answered honestly, "Probably not." In stark contrast to her departure less than two months prior, the airports were busy and her flight home was full.

When she arrived home, Stacy had to stay in mandatory quarantine for 14 days—time in isolation from her daughter, family and friends, time to decompress from all she had just seen and heard, time to make sure that she hadn't been infected with the virus she had been helping others fight. Her first order of business was food, so someone volunteered to drop off her favorite tacos and beer. On her first night home, and for the first time in almost 2 months, she played with her kittens and slept in her own bed.

Over the next few days, Stacy reacclimated to her surroundings and adjusted into "normalcy." Suddenly, in the comfort of her own home, she didn't have to over-think everything she touched and when she washed her hands. After the hyper-vigilance of the last 50 days, it took some time to adjust into the comfort and routine of her own space.

Stacy describes re-entry:

*"It's been hard. I'm really struggling. I miss NYC. I miss my hospital. I miss the nursing agency staff. I miss the hospital staff. I regret leaving when I did, and I feel like I should have stayed longer. When I watch videos about my time there or see pictures, it brings back the sights and the sounds and the smells so vividly. I love what we accomplished there, and, as hard as it was, I knew every day that we were making a difference. I knew what we were doing would be a part of history. Going from this profound sense of purpose to having to isolate in quarantine and do "nothing" is very traumatic. It feels unnat-ural. I have trouble focusing. My normally tidy apartment is messy and I can't seem to get back into the same routines I had before I left. I lose things like my wallet and car keys.*

*I forget things. I didn't have to keep up with all those little things for 50 days, and now it's like relearning a habit I had somehow forgotten. Washing dishes, doing laundry, sitting down and sitting still to watch TV or read a book...all those tasks are proving to be difficult. I have nightmares, and I am admittedly impatient about things that don't seem to be important. I always compare the relevance or importance of things to the situation in NYC, and for obvious reasons, people who weren't there don't understand that. I find my brain wanting to do things, be social, etc., but my body has different plans. I usually have about 1-2 good focused alert hours a day. After that, everything just gets fuzzy and I get tired, and I'm ready to retreat back into isolation and not deal with anything or anyone else."*

There are thousands of healthcare workers who ran into NYC to help patients and fight COVID and, like Stacy Ellis, they are all heroes who chose to show up and answer a call. Through this experience, a kinship of NY COVID nurses has emerged. These women and men will forever be bound by their compassion for humankind and their willingness to put themselves at risk to face the unknown. Like Stacy, many of the nurses who deployed stayed much longer than their contracts called for, all for their own various and personal reasons. Their shared experiences in NY made them family—brothers and sisters for life, no matter where their journeys take them. There's no telling how many individual lives they collectively saved.

Despite her answer to the hospital staff of probably not going back, Stacy knows now that she would return to NY in a heartbeat. It's likely that many of the other nurses would do the same. This family of nurses held each other up, recognizing that if a similar crisis were to happen in their own towns or cities, that people, just like them, would come to help as well. This compassionate belief in the goodness of humankind, even in the face of the worst conditions and with the sickest of patients, is the spirit that will move us forward, because each of us can make a difference to someone, even if it's one person. To that end, Stacy referenced "The Starfish Parable:"

> *One day, an old man was walking along a beach that was littered with thousands of starfish that had been washed ashore by the high tide. As he walked, he came upon*

*a young boy who was eagerly throwing the starfish back into the ocean, one by one.*

*Puzzled, the man looked at the boy and asked what he was doing. Without looking up from his task, the boy simply replied, "I'm saving these starfish, Sir".*

*The old man chuckled aloud, "Son, there are thousands of starfish and only one of you. What difference can you make?"*

*The boy picked up a starfish, gently tossed it into the water and turning to the man, said, "I made a difference to that one!"*

My friend and my derby sister, Stacy Ellis, House of Pain, is a hero. She and her family of NY COVID nurses chose to show up when humanity called. They chose to make a difference, to one person, to many, to all. These heroes helped all of us survive the "dash" between what was and what will be.

While the pandemic is far from over, the urgency in NYC has subsided, and there is an attempt to find a new normal, where people can cautiously and safely live their lives. Given the continued lack of information and the ever-rising COVID numbers, there are some important takeaways from Stacy's story for all of us to consider. These are not partisan issues, but, rather, matters of science and care for our essential workers.

Please consider these thoughts with an open mind, keeping at the forefront that these are the words of a frontline COVID nurse:

1.  The federal government's response to COVID was disappointing, including the ever-changing "PPE Minimum Requirements." There was a failure to provide the bare minimum of PPE to keep us safe. For the first 3 weeks, each nurse was given one N95 in a brown paper sack with direction to reuse it for 5 days. This is not how N95s are intended to be used. Before COVID they were always considered single-use masks. I worry about the long-term effects for all of us from wearing reused N95s, for 12+ hours a day, for up to five days at a time.

2.  There are lasting physical and psychological effects that caregivers are experiencing related to our relief efforts. Many of my fellow nurses have reported extremely difficult transitions back to home life, anxiety, nightmares, and symptoms similar to PTSD. I am thankful our agency has given us resources to reach out to crisis counselors. All care workers should be provided the same resources.

3. I ask, hope and pray that our government finds better ways to protect all healthcare providers, and does more to recognize their contributions. If healthcare workers can't protect themselves and trust that we will be taken care of when we run to the call of a pandemic, who will answer the call the next time?

4. To my family and friends: promise me when this all becomes manageable again, you will do one thing to demand answers and change. Pick one issue. *One.* There are so many issues we must sort out. Pick one and place it in your heart and mind and seek answers and fight for change.

Don't let this all be for nothing. We are better than this.

# About Candy

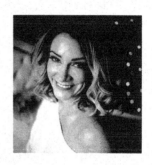

 C ANDY LEIGH LIVES IN SOUTH-eastern Wisconsin. She is the president and owner of Candy Leigh Coaching, LLC. She spent the majority of her career in the financial services industry for a Fortune 500 company, most notably developing diversity and inclusion leadership programs. Candy also spent many years consulting with and coaching sales executives and leaders across the nation.

After a successful corporate career Candy branched out on her own. She decided to pursue her dream of writing and coaching and advocating for individuals. As a coach, Candy's mission is to help all individuals to stand in their truth and live authentically. She believes that when we can honestly share our authentic selves in safe spaces, not only do we show up as better employees/spouses/partners, we ultimately open ourselves up to leading more fulfilling lives.

Candy is the mother of three children and two long-haired miniature dachshunds. When she is not with her family, she is often traveling to visit her "framily" (friends who are family). She is a retired rollergirl, former triathlete and half-marathoner. Candy is an avid yoga enthusiast, Double Stuf Oreo lover, and self-proclaimed goddess of her own untamed and beautifully imperfect life.

Candy's first book, *Finding Life In Between*, is available now on Amazon.com.

# About Stacy

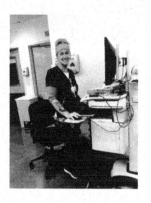

Stacy is a Registered Nurse in San Antonio, TX. Nursing has been her passion for over ten years. She currently works with adults with developmental disabilities. Stacy enjoys making a difference for people who aren't always able to advocate for themselves. She hopes to further her nursing education and become a psychiatric nurse practitioner.

Stacy's nursing philosophy is the Starfish Parable. When the tasks at hand seem overwhelming and daunting, making a difference to "that one" is the place to start and helps guide her nursing practice.

When she isn't working, she enjoys Texas country music, reading, and listening to true crime podcasts.

# Blessed, Stressed, but Still Flying

Maureen Cavanaugh

I N MID-DECEMBER OF 2019, I EARNED MY FLIGHT AT-
tendant wings at my dream airline. I packed my life
into my car and drove 14 hours to my new home base in
Chicago where I found an apartment and started building a new life. I was a new hire, bottom of the flight
attendant food chain, flying reserve trips but so eagerly
optimistic about the future. Within a matter of months,
the COVID-19 pandemic had turned the entire airline
industry on its head.

There were new route cancellations each week.
Grounded airplanes filled up the hangars. Rumors circulated about furloughs. I was starting a new career, I
wasn't making a lot of money, and I had no job senior-
ity. It was a scary time to be new.

Each day a million thoughts ran through my head:
*When will we hear the bad news from the company?
How long can this last? How long can we go on like
this, flying empty planes? What should I do with my
apartment lease? Will I need to find a new job? A tem-
porary job? Who is even hiring right now? What if
I have to move all over again? Will the government
give the airlines another bailout? How can I plan my
life more than six months in advance when my future
is hanging on by a thread?*

I never felt so many different voices shouting in my
head at once. I felt so blessed, so incredibly fortunate
to still have a job. But I felt overwhelmed with the

stress of what was coming next. In the end, I realized there was no point in worrying about the future. The only thing I could do was keep pinning on my wings and flying until there was nothing left to be flown.

With each trip that I flew, I could see the pandemic slowly overtaking life. I worked a trip to Japan in January on a flight that was nearly full; social distancing was not even a concept yet. By February, passengers had started showing up with masks and wipes. Some people thought it was a bit extreme. In March, the White House declared a national emergency, and I worked a busy flight to St. Thomas the next week. That flight was filled with families going on spring break despite stay-at-home orders. By the following week, the planes were completely empty. A lone passenger every ten rows. In April, I started wearing a mask to work because they were now company approved. Not long after that, the masks were required, along with temperature checks. Airports were nothing but ghost towns with plastic-wrapped restaurant chairs and elevator music drifting through the halls.

We started handing out Purell wipes during boarding. We distributed sealed drinks and sealed food in flight. No ice, no coffee, no liquor. We limited our contact with passengers. It all seemed to change so suddenly. A few months ago, I was in training learning how to pour wine and use a silver tray in business class.

Now, the best service I could give a passenger was staying as far away from them as possible.

When people ask me if I'm afraid of contracting the virus, my answer is always no.

Flight attendants have been so exposed from day one that the thought of losing my job is more worrying to me. Flight attendants have a huge sense of pride in what they do. Many of us have worked so hard to get to where we are. We wouldn't go to yearly training or put up with cranky passengers, delays, and tumultuous schedules if we didn't love it. For many, it is a lifestyle, a mindset, a community, the only job they have ever known.

As much as things seem to be looking up, business is still unpredictable in the airline industry. Particularly for new hires like me, our jobs are uncertain. Demand remains lower than ever. With so many country entry restrictions, airlines struggle making money in the international market. The initial round of government bailout money to supply employee payroll will run out eventually.

In September, I joined many other junior flight attendants at my company to march in Washington, DC, urging Congress to pass another bill to extend our payroll support program. It was that or collect unemployment. We were met with overwhelming support from our company and union. We marched around

Capitol Hill with masks and signs, demanding action from our country's leaders. Despite our actions, it seems unlikely Congress will pass another bill for the airlines, at least not before furloughs go into effect. Time is running out and I may have to hang up my wings and find another job for now.

So, you may get on a plane soon. It might be the first flight you've taken since COVID broke out. You may be wearing a mask and the middle seats may be empty for social distancing. And I may not be there. I may be off doing something else, waiting for my job to become available again. I may be finishing a bachelor's degree or learning French online or finally cooking all those recipes I saved on Pinterest.

But just know that we, flight attendants, are so happy you are here. We have spent so many days cooped up at home on company leave or sitting around waiting for a flight assignment that isn't coming.

We miss telling you how to open the bathroom door or apologizing that we're out of Diet Coke. We miss asking you to kindly take your yoga out of the galley area. We miss overstuffed bins and people traveling with too many bags.

We miss those people who order a Jack and Coke at six in the morning. We miss the captain getting on the PA system and saying, "There is heavy air traffic heading into New York. We'll be waiting here for a while."

We miss the days when our biggest concerns were chicken or beef and whether the hotel at the layover was downtown. We miss breaking our nails opening soda cans and burning our fingertips on the galley ovens. We miss repeating the same information from one person to the next because no one is listening.

We miss jumpseat heart-to-hearts with coworkers we just met but feel like family already. We miss seeing kids and first-time fliers look out the window on an approach to New York City. We miss the long, long TSA security lines. We miss the hugs and tears and 'welcome home' signs at airport arrivals.

If you do get on a plane in 2021, or whenever things are back to normal, know that we are happy to have you here. We value your business. It is our pleasure to fly you to your destination.

# About Maureen

M AUREEN CAVANAUGH DEVeloped a passion for traveling in high school, earning the senior award of most likely to become a flight attendant. She fulfilled that dream at the age of 19, flying for a regional airline based in Washington, 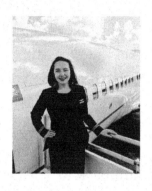 DC. She flew for three years on tiny 70-seater jets before transitioning to a major airline in late 2019. She is one of 6,920 flight attendants at her company that were involuntarily furloughed in October 2020 as a result of the COVID-19 pandemic. While she is granted recall rights when market demand returns, she has dedicated her time off to finishing her Bachelor of Arts in Communications. She hopes to pursue work in digital media, marketing, or public relations while waiting to return back to flying. Maureen is from the Washington, DC area and currently does not know where to call home. Follow her travels and job experiences @maureencvngh on Instagram and Twitter and at her blog thebattered passport.wordpress.com.

# Faced With Uncertainties

Emmy Li

W HEN COVID STARTED TO SPREAD THROUGHOUT China, no one guessed that it would become a nationwide pandemic in the States. We were first in denial as we watched things unfold from a distance, then things quickly began to escalate. In mid to late February, the hospitalization rates in New York City hospitals slowly began to rise. COVID patients were coming into our ICU's with respiratory issues, needing ventilators and critical care attention. Treatment of these patients was our primary concern and protecting ourselves as healthcare workers, was our secondary concern. COVID-19 brought so much uncertainty and fear because of how new the pandemic was to all of us. It made healthcare workers question if the hospitalizations were ever going to stabilize, if we were going to have enough protective equipment and, if our family and friends were going to be safe. We walked into work every day knowing that we were exposing ourselves to this virus that everyone else was trying to get away from.

Regardless of whether we saw this coming or not, the truth is that we were not prepared. We are currently at war with an invisible enemy that finds and attacks the weakest amongst us.

As I reflect back to that time, I realize that this is the reason why I became a nurse. I am drawn to the desire to help and serve. Most importantly, I am proud to be able to make a difference in my patients' care and to be where I am needed the most.

The beginning of the COVID crisis was very strenuous because my first COVID patient was my own grandfather.

He was an 85-year-old lung cancer survivor who never smoked and was for the most part healthy. I didn't live at home but I would occasionally visit a few times a month. When my mom told me that my grandpa was not feeling well, the worst thoughts started coming to mind. As an ICU nurse, I couldn't help but to think that way. Grandpa was presenting early signs and symptoms of COVID when I saw him. I tried every supportive care treatment possible but, in the end, it wasn't enough. He needed medical attention, but he kept refusing to go to the hospital.

My ridiculous and desperate thoughts led me to think of bringing home the hospital so that I could start treating him. Realistically, I explained to him his condition and the importance of getting treated at the hospital but he kept telling me that he was fine and that he didn't need to go. During further inquiry, I found out that he didn't want to go to the hospital because, in his words, "If I go to the hospital, I am going to come out with more problems."

Eventually, I made the decision to take matters into my own hands and called an ambulance. It was the better option for the rest of my family.

If grandpa did have the virus, then everyone else was at risk.

When the medics arrived, they put grandpa on the monitor and it showed that his heart rhythm was unstable. Unfortunately they had no medications to give on hand, so we were in agreement that he needed the right treatment at the hospital. Grandpa again resisted on going. The medics had to physically restrain him and take him into the ambulance. Grandpa used every breath and energy he had to fight against us. I held his hand on the ambulance and tried to comfort him but he was still uneasy.

I was scared of what was going on in the hospital because I saw it. I feared what would happen behind closed doors since I wouldn't be able to visit.

I feared that he was COVID positive.

When we arrived at the hospital, my emotions heightened because I had to discuss resuscitation and intubation of my grandpa, if the occasion presented itself, with the physician. After a long discussion with my grandpa and the medical team led him to decide that DNR/DNI was what he wanted. This proved to be even more of a challenge when I had to be the mediator amongst my family. Speaking about this decision to the rest of the family was not easy because they were all against his wishes. They constantly said things like "this is not what Grandpa wants, he is just confused," and although it was extremely difficult to sign and accept, I knew he was not confused at all and that it was what he wanted.

Grandpa was admitted into the hospital Saturday night. Each day became more and more uncertain because visitation was prohibited. Each day felt extremely long, just waiting to hear his progress. Every day I would call at least three times, but only would be able to reach the medical team once.

On the afternoon of Tuesday March 24th, 2020, I was finally able to get in touch with the medical team. I asked about his overall condition, what kind of oxygen he was on, his vitals and his labs. All the information provided to me told me that he was doing okay.

Minutes later the same physician assistant called to tell me that he had passed.

I questioned him furiously saying, "You just told me he was okay, were you not watching him? How could this happen?"

His only answer was, "It's COVID."

And just like that he was gone. It was hard for any of us to grasp. We were all in denial, thinking how could this be?

COVID took away many lives. What hurts even more was that many died alone. Even after his passing, circumstances still didn't allow us to see him. If I could see him again, I would say, "Grandpa, you don't need to fight anymore. You can go peacefully. Thank you for everything you did for me and the family. I will always remember you. We will meet again."

I know in my heart that Grandpa fought to take each breath until the very end because that is who I remember him to be, a man with a strong head on his shoulders and a hard foot on the ground.

Dealing with Grandpa's death was extremely difficult. It drained me. The need for support felt greater but was hard to obtain during this time of social distancing. That gave me some time to reflect. I knew that I couldn't let it mentally bring me down.

I pledged to continue to take care of COVID patients because I knew they needed me. These patients needed someone to take care of them like family and as weird as it sounded, taking care of them also helped me to cope with my loss.

I worked with a strong ICU team at my hospital I was previously at. Our manager worked with us from the beginning, with the intentions of protecting us and our patients. My coworkers raised funds to provide us with enough protective equipment and, with all these precautions, my coworkers still got sick. As the number of call-outs increased, the demand for critical care attention also increased. My nursing coworkers and I were floating to newly created COVID units in our hospital, gowned and masked up for eleven hours straight.

We all had at least four to five patients during each shift, while precepting other nurses in critical care.

Our patients were in severe acute respiratory distress syndrome and septic. They needed to be intubated and to be placed on multiple IV medications to maintain stability. These COVID patients were all high risks to code and the end results of COVID were multisystem organ failures leading to death. It was hard to fight off this virus without enough medical knowledge, but we tried everything we could as we learned and adjusted to the new information every day.

While I was still healing from my open wound, my father started developing signs of COVID one week later. At 76, my father has a history of diabetes, hypertension, and hyperlipidemia. This caused me so much fear because it felt like I was back in the same boat. He said he felt fine, but he didn't look fine. Over time, he developed shortness of breath so I brought him to the hospital where I worked because I knew I could at least see him there.

At this point, I felt like I was living in COVID. My partner had COVID. Half my family was presenting with symptoms. My dad was admitted into the hospital. On top of this, I still tried to focus on fighting for the lives of my COVID patients. I checked on my dad in between breaks and when I was off the clock. With each visit there was progress which assured me a road to recovery. And true to my thoughts, my father started feeling better just a few days after being admitted. My dad made it out as a COVID survivor. I was very thankful to the medical team that took care of him.

When I reflect back on these times, the one memory that really touches me was when I sat at my father's bedside in the hospital. He said to me, "In all these years, I never got a chance to see where you work. Now that I am sick, I am finally able to see it." I responded by assuring him that it was okay, and then we took a picture together.

We are learning something new about this virus every day, but every day we are also losing more lives. This has brought down everyone's spirit. I wanted to do something for my unit to improve morale, but I wasn't sure what to do. Eventually, I reached out to community restaurants to see if we could get donations to health care workers. To my surprise, I received a few responses which led me to building more connections. During this time, I saw the love from our community and how so many people were willing to help. I worked with Jessica Fields who organized Meals for Brooklyn Healthcare Heroes on GoFundMe. She worked with me to make sure that our ICU was getting food daily until the funds ran out. I also connected with COVID supporters, @covidersupporters, on social media platforms who organized and worked with companies that distributed wellness products. This generosity showed me that even in the darkest times, there is still that shining light in humanity.

It was a long two month battle of COVID. During this time, it was nice to get the help from the travel nurses who came from all over to help. The sky started clearing when our COVID admissions were trending down. The workload became somewhat normal again.

A few of our patients recovered. Those who made it out of ICU needed some recovery time to gain their strength back from the shock to their body. They were one step closer to go home and see their family once again. Each discharge and survival story brought an inner state of fulfillment and was worth celebrating for. Each felt like an accomplishment for us to see that we were able to make a difference.

I continued to work in ICU as a nurse a bit longer after the surge, but then transitioned into working as a nurse practitioner at a COVID testing site. Screening the community and teaching preventative measures are the best ways to prevent the spread. I found myself making a difference during this pandemic in every way I can.

It's been a tough year. COVID took away a lot. It took away our loved ones and our piece of mind. But at the end of it all, I find joy in what I do. I am living out my purpose to help and care for others. This is my superhero power. I don't wear capes, I wear scrubs.

# About Emmy

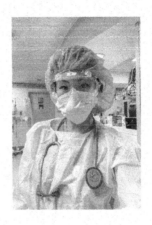

EMMY LI IS AMERICAN BORN, Asian-America healthcare worker. She was raised by her grandparents in Shang-hai, China and was later brought up by parents with strict traditional values. At an early age, she knew she wanted to work in a profession where she is able to live out her purpose of helping and make an impact on others. She is currently working as a nurse practitioner for NYC COVID testing site. Emmy devotes her time to taking care of others and is expanding her interest into becoming a Psych NP to help those who face mental health challenges.

# About The Unapologetic Voice House

T HE UNAPOLOGETIC VOICE HOUSE IS AN INDEPENDENT publishing house based in Arizona. We have a passion for stories and storytellers.

We operate much like an agency with a talented team of editors, designers and managers supporting our authors.

Check out our titles at www.theunapologeticvoicehouse.com